C000133519

Keto Chaffle Cookbook for Your Daily Meals

50 recipes to cook for any occasion

Catherine Willis

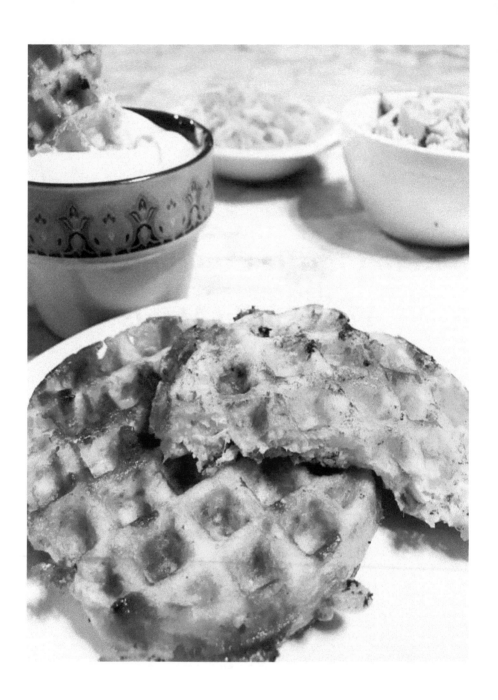

© Copyright 2021 - All rights reserved.

The content contained within this book may not be reproduced, duplicated or transmitted without direct written permission from the author or the publisher.

Under no circumstances will any blame or legal responsibility be held against the publisher, or author, for any damages, reparation, or monetary loss due to the information contained within this book. Either directly or indirectly.

Legal Notice:

This book is copyright protected. This book is only for personal use. You cannot amend, distribute, sell, use, quote or paraphrase any part, or the content within this book, without the consent of the author or publisher.

Disclaimer Notice:

Please note the information contained within this document is for educational and entertainment purposes only. All effort has been executed to present accurate, up to date, and reliable, complete information. No warranties of any kind are declared or implied. Readers acknowledge that the author is not engaging in the rendering of legal, financial, medical or professional advice. The content within this book has been derived from various sources. Please consult a licensed professional before attempting any techniques outlined in this book.

By reading this document, the reader agrees that under no circumstances is the author responsible for any losses, direct or indirect, which are incurred as a result of the use of information contained within this document, including, but not limited to, — errors, omissions, or inaccuracies.

Table of Contents

1. Cream Cake Chaffle 7

2. Almond Butter Chaffles 9

3. Layered Chaffles 11

4. Simple Mozzarella Chaffles 12

5. Cream Mini-chaffles 14

6. Raspberry Chaffles 16

7. Lemon Chaffles... 18

8. Chocolate Chip Waffles... 20

9. Pumpkin & Psyllium Husk Chaffles 22

10. Blackberry Chaffles... 24

11. Pumpkin Cream Cheese Chaffles 26

12. Cinnamon Pecan Waffles....................................... 28

13. Chaffle Glazed with Raspberry 30

14. Oreo Keto Chaffles.. 32

15. Cinnamon Sugar Waffles....................................... 34

16. Cream Cheese Chaffles 36

17. Mozzarella & Butter Chaffles................................. 38

18. Pumpkin Pecan Waffles... 40

19. Chocolate Cream Chaffles...................................... 42

20. Blueberry Cinnamon Chaffles 44

21. Gingerbread Chaffle 47

22. Chocolate Whipping Cream Chaffles.................................. 49

23. Almond Flour Waffles 51

24. Strawberry cake Chaffles 53

25. Cream Cheese & Butter Chaffles................................ 55

26. Chocolate Cherry Chaffles 58

27. Coconut & Walnut Chaffles 60

28. Chocolate Chaffles 62

29. Chocolate Chips & Whipping Cream Chaffles 64

30. Spiced Pumpkin Waffles... 66

31. Vanilla Chaffle 68

32. Banana Nut Chaffle 70

33. Chocolate Chips Pumpkin Waffles 72

34. Oreo Chaffles 74

35. Whipping Cream Pumpkin Chaffles.........................77

36. Chocolate Vanilla Chaffles...................................... 79

37. Churro Waffles...81

38. Chocolate Chips Lemon Chaffles........................... 83

39. Mocha Chaffles 85

40. Carrot Chaffles... 87

41. Yogurt Chaffles 90

42. Chocolate Peanut Butter Chaffles.......................... 92

43. Ube Waffles With Ice Cream 94

44. Berries Chaffles...96

45. Cinnamon Swirl Waffles..98

46. Chocolate Cream Cheese Chaffles 101

47. Colby Jack Chaffles..103

48. Chaffle Birthday Cake..104

49. Chaffle Churros..107

50. Strawberry Chaffles 109

Cream Cake Chaffle

Preparation time : 8 minutes

Cooking Time : 12 Minutes

Servings : 2

INGREDIENTS :

Chaffle

4 oz cream cheese, softened

4 eggs

4 tbsp coconut flour

1 tbsp almond flour

1 ½ tsp baking powder

1 tbsp butter, softened

1 tsp vanilla extract

½ tsp cinnamon

1 tbsp sweetener

1 tbsp shredded coconut, colored and unsweetened

1 tbsp walnuts, chopped

Italian Cream Frosting

2 oz cream cheese, softened

2 tbsp butter, room temperature

2 tbsp sweetener

½ tsp vanilla

DIRECTIONS :

1. Preheat your waffle maker and add ¼ of the
2. Cook for 3 minutes and repeat the process until you have 4 chaffles.
3. Remove and set aside.
4. In the meantime, start making your frosting by mixing all the
5. Stir until you have a smooth and creamy mixture.
6. Cool, frost the cake and enjoy.

NUTRITION :

Calories 127 Kcal ; Fats: 10 g ; Carbs: 5.5 g ; Protein: 7 g

Almond Butter Chaffles

Preparation time : 5 minutes

Cooking Time : 10 Minutes

Servings : 2

INGREDIENTS :

    1 large organic egg, beaten

    1/3 cup Mozzarella cheese, shredded

    1 tablespoon Erythritol

    2 tablespoons almond butter

    1 teaspoon organic vanilla extract

DIRECTIONS :

1. Preheat a mini waffle iron and then grease it.
2. In a medium bowl, place all **INGREDIENTS** and with a fork, mix until well combined.
3. Put a portion of the mixture into preheated waffle iron and cook for about 5 minutes or until golden brown.
4. Repeat with the remaining mixture.
5. Serve warm.

NUTRITION :

Calories: 153Net Carb: 2gFat: 12.3gSaturated Fat: 2gCarbohydrates: 3.Dietary Fiber: 1.6g Sugar: 1.2gProtein: 7.9 g

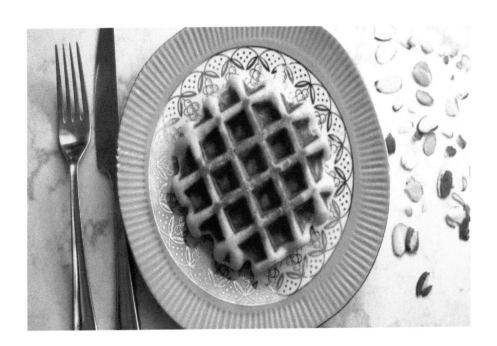

Layered Chaffles

Preparation time : 5 minutes

Cooking Time : 10 Minutes

Servings : 2

INGREDIENTS :

> 1 organic egg, beaten and divided
>
> ½ cup cheddar cheese, shredded and divided
>
> Pinch of salt

DIRECTIONS :

1. Preheat a mini waffle iron and then grease it.
2. Place about 1/8 cup of cheese in the bottom of the waffle iron and top with half of the beaten egg.
3. Now, place 1/8 cup of cheese on top and cook for about 4–5 minutes.
4. Repeat with the remaining cheese and egg.
5. Serve warm.

NUTRITION :

Calories 145 Net Carbs 0.5 g Total Fat 11.g Saturated Fat 6.6 gCholesterol 112 mg Sodium 284 g Total Carbs 0.5 gFiber 0 g Sugar 0.3 gProtein 9.8 g

Simple Mozzarella Chaffles

Preparation time : 5 minutes

Cooking Time : 8 Minutes

Servings : 2

INGREDIENTS :

> ½ cup mozzarella cheese, shredded
>
> 1 large organic egg
>
> 2 tablespoons blanched almond flour
>
> ¼ teaspoon organic baking powder
>
> 2–3 drops liquid stevia

DIRECTIONS :

1. Preheat a mini waffle iron and then grease it.
2. In a medium bowl, put all ingredients and with a fork, mix until well combined. Put a portion of the mixture into preheated waffle iron and cook for about 3–4 minutes.
3. Repeat with the remaining mixture.
4. Serve warm.

NUTRITION :

Calories 98 Net Carbs 1.4 g Total Fat 7.1 g Saturated Fat 1.8 gCholesterol 97 mgSodium 81 mg Total Carbs 2.2 gFiber 0.8 g Sugar 0.2 gProtein 6.7 g

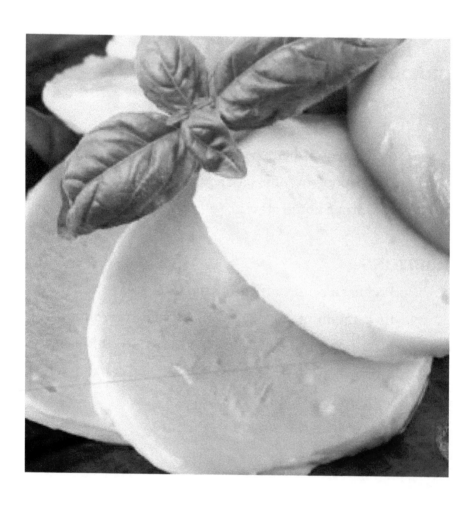

Cream Mini-chaffles

Preparation time : 5 minutes

Cooking Time : 10 Minutes

Servings : 2

INGREDIENTS :

      2 tsp coconut flour

      4 tsp swerve/monk fruit

      ¼ tsp baking powder

      1 egg

      1 oz cream cheese

      ½ tsp vanilla extract

DIRECTIONS :

1. Turn on the waffle maker to heat and oil it with cooking spray.
2. Mix swerve/monk fruit, coconut flour, and baking powder in a small mixing bowl.
3. Add cream cheese, egg, vanilla extract, and whisk until well-combined.
4. Add batter into the waffle maker and cook for 3-minutes, until golden brown.
5. Serve with your favorite toppings.

NUTRITION :

Carbs: 4 g;Fat: g;Protein: 2 g;Calories: 73

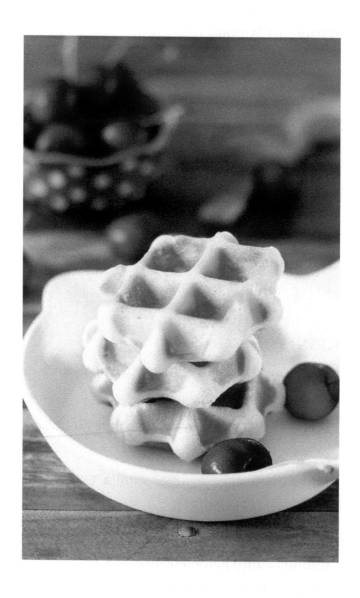

Raspberry Chaffles

Preparation time : 5 minutes

Cooking Time : 5 Minutes

Servings : 5

INGREDIENTS :

    4 Tbsp almond flour

    4 large eggs

    2⅓ cup shredded mozzarella cheese

    1 tsp vanilla extract

    1 Tbsp erythritol sweetener

    1½ tsp baking powder

    ½ cup raspberries

DIRECTIONS :

1. Turn on the waffle maker to heat and oil it with cooking spray.
2. Mix almond flour, sweetener, and baking powder in a bowl.
3. Add cheese, eggs, and vanilla extract, and mix until well-combined.
4. Add 1 portion of batter to the waffle maker and spread it evenly. Close and cook for 3-minutes, or until golden.

5. Repeat until remaining batter is used.

6. Serve with raspberries.

NUTRITION :

Carbs: 5 g;Fat: 11 g;Protein: 24 g;Calories: 300

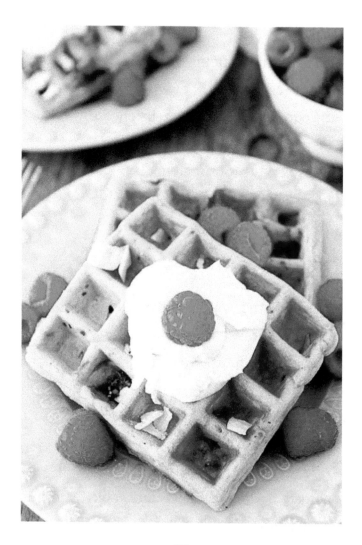

Lemon Chaffles

Preparation time : 5 minutes

Cooking Time : 10 Minutes

Servings : 2

INGREDIENTS :

      1 organic egg, beaten

      1 ounce cream cheese, softened

      2 tablespoons almond flour

      1 tablespoon fresh lemon juice

      2 teaspoons Erythritol

      ½ teaspoon fresh lemon zest, grated

      ¼ teaspoon organic baking powder

      Pinch of salt

      ½ teaspoon powdered Erythritol

  DIRECTIONS :

1. Preheat a mini waffle iron and then grease it.
2. In a bowl, place all ingredients except the powdered Erythritol and beat until well combined.
3. Put a portion of the mixture into preheated waffle iron and cook for about 5 minutes or until golden brown.
4. Repeat with the remaining mixture.

5. Serve warm with the sprinkling of powdered Erythritol.

NUTRITION :

Calories: 129Net Carb: 1.2gFat: 10.9gSaturated Fat: 4.1gCarbohydrates: 2.4gDietary Fiber: 0.8g Sugar: 0.Protein: 3.9 g

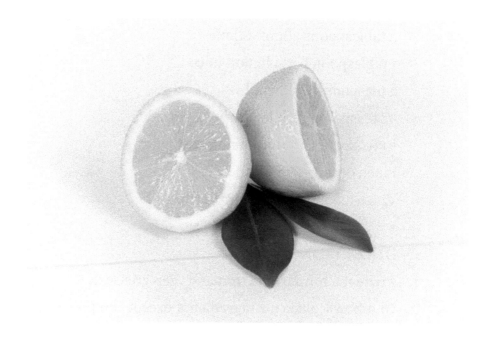

Chocolate Chip Waffles

Preparation time : 8 minutes

Servings : 1

Cooking Time :6 Minutes

INGREDIENTS :

    1 egg

    1 tsp coconut flour

    1 tsp sweetener

    ½ tsp vanilla extract

    ¼ cup heavy whipping cream, for serving

    ½ cup almond milk ricotta, finely shredded

    2 tbsp sugar-free chocolate chips

DIRECTIONS :

1. Preheat your mini waffle iron.
2. Mix the egg, coconut flour, vanilla, and sweetener. Whisk together with a fork.
3. Stir in the almond milk ricotta.
4. Introduce half of the batter into the waffle iron and dot with a pinch of chocolate chips.
5. Close the waffle iron and cook for minutes.
6. Repeat with remaining batter.
7. Serve hot with the whipped cream.

NUTRITION :

Calories per **Serving s** : 304 Kcal ; Fats:16 g ; Carbs: 7 g ;
Protein: 3 g

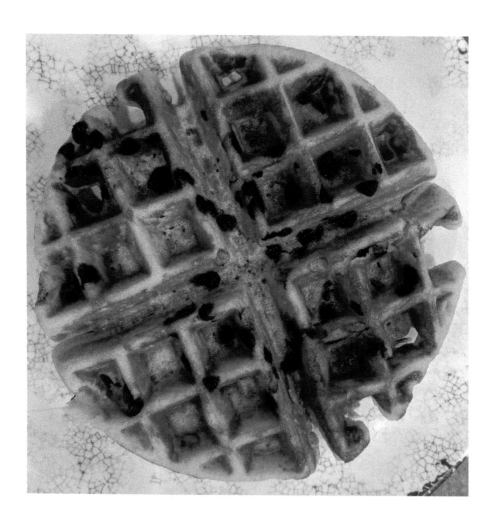

Pumpkin & Psyllium Husk Chaffles

Preparation time : 8 minutes

Cooking Time : 16 Minutes

Servings : 2

INGREDIENTS :

2 organic eggs

½ cup mozzarella cheese, shredded

1 tablespoon homemade pumpkin puree

2 teaspoons Erythritol

½ teaspoon psyllium husk powder

1/3 teaspoon ground cinnamon

Pinch of salt

½ teaspoon organic vanilla extract

DIRECTIONS :

1. Preheat a mini waffle iron and then grease it.
2. In a bowl, place all ingredients and beat until well combined.
3. Place ¼ of the mixture into preheated waffle iron and cook for about 4 minutes or until golden brown.
4. Repeat with the remaining mixture.
5. Serve warm.

NUTRITION :

Calories: 4et Carb: 0.6gFat: 2.8gSaturated Fat: 1.1gCarbohydrates: 0.8gDietary Fiber: 0.2g Sugar: 0.4gProtein: 3.9g

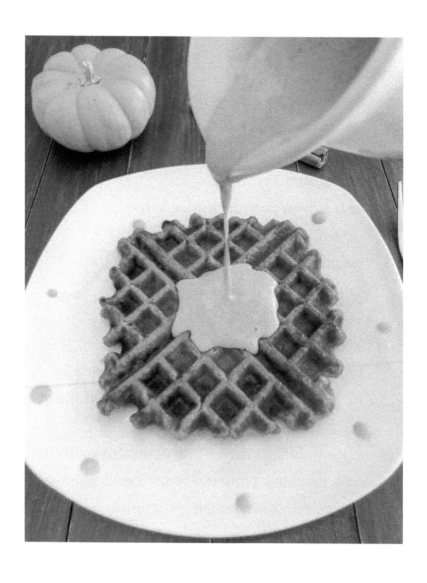

Blackberry Chaffles

Preparation time : 5 minutes

Cooking Time : 8 Minutes

Servings : 2

INGREDIENTS :

> 1 organic egg, beaten
>
> 1/3 cup Mozzarella cheese, shredded
>
> 1 teaspoon cream cheese, softened
>
> 1 teaspoon coconut flour
>
> ¼ teaspoon organic baking powder
>
> ¾ teaspoon powdered Erythritol
>
> ¼ teaspoon ground cinnamon
>
> ¼ teaspoon organic vanilla extract
>
> Pinch of salt
>
> 1 tablespoon fresh blackberries

DIRECTIONS :

1. Preheat a mini waffle iron and then grease it.
2. In a bowl, place all **INGREDIENTS** except for blackberries and beat until well combined.
3. Fold in the blackberries.

4. Put a portion of the mixture into preheated waffle iron and cook for about minutes or until golden brown.
5. Repeat with the remaining mixture.
6. Serve warm.

NUTRITION :

Calories: 121Net Carb: 2.Fat: 7.5gSaturated Fat: 3.3gCarbohydrates: 4.5gDietary Fiber: 1.8g Sugar: 0.9gProtein: 8.9g

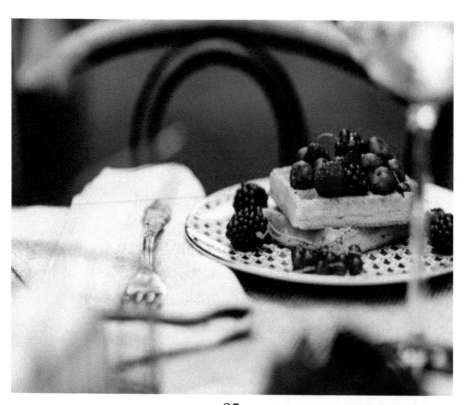

Pumpkin Cream Cheese Chaffles

Preparation time : 5 minutes

Cooking Time : 10 Minutes

Servings : 2

INGREDIENTS :

     1 organic egg, beaten

     ½ cup Mozzarella cheese, shredded

     1½ tablespoon sugar-free pumpkin puree

     2 teaspoons heavy cream

     1 teaspoon cream cheese, softened

     1 tablespoon almond flour

     1 tablespoon Erythritol

     ½ teaspoon pumpkin pie spice

     ½ teaspoon organic baking powder

     1 teaspoon organic vanilla extract

DIRECTIONS :

1. Preheat a mini waffle iron and then grease it.
2. In a medium bowl, place all ingredients and with a fork, mix until well combined.
3. Put a portion of the mixture into preheated waffle iron and cook for about 5 minutes or until golden brown.

4. Repeat with the remaining mixture.

5. Serve warm.

NUTRITION :

Calories: 110Net Carb: 2.5gFat: 4.3gSaturated Fat: 1gCarbohydrates: 3.3gDietary Fiber: 0.8g Sugar: 1gProtein: 5.2g

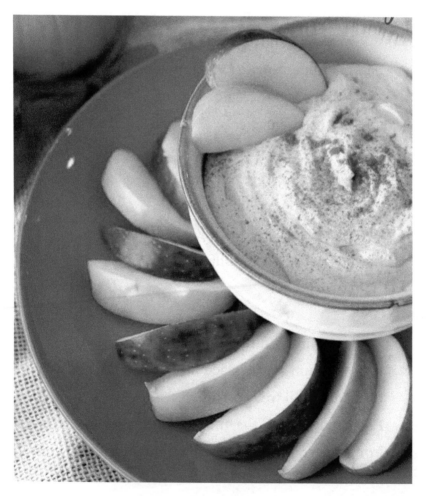

Cinnamon Pecan Waffles

Preparation time : 5 minutes

Servings : 1

Cooking Time : 40 Minutes

INGREDIENTS :

      1 Tbsp butter

      1 egg

      ½ tsp vanilla

      2 Tbsp almond flour

      1 Tbsp coconut flour

      ⅛ tsp baking powder

      1 Tbsp monk fruit

      For the crumble:

      ½ tsp cinnamon

      1 Tbsp melted butter

      1 tsp monk fruit

      1 Tbsp chopped pecans

DIRECTIONS :

1. Turn on the waffle maker to heat and oil it with cooking spray.
2. Melt butter in a bowl, then mix in the egg and vanilla.

3. Mix in remaining chaffle ingredients.
4. Combine crumble ingredients in a separate bowl.
5. Introduce half of the chaffle mix into the waffle maker. Top with half of the crumble mixture.
6. Cook for 5 minutes, or until done.
7. Repeat with the other half of the batter.

NUTRITION :

Carbs: g;Fat: 35 g;Protein: 10 g;Calories: 391

Chaffle Glazed with Raspberry

Preparation time : 5 minutes

Servings : 1

Cooking Time : 5 Minutes

INGREDIENTS :

Donut Chaffle ingredients:

1 egg

¼ cup mozzarella cheese, shredded

2 tsp cream cheese, softened

1 tsp sweetener

1tsp almond flour

½ tsp baking powder

20 drops glazed donut flavoring

Raspberry Jelly Filling:

¼ cup raspberries

1 tsp chia seeds

1 tsp confectioners' sweetener

Donut Glaze:

1 tsp powdered sweetener

Heavy whipping cream

DIRECTIONS :

1. Spray your waffle maker with cooking oil and add the butter mixture into the waffle maker.
2. Cook for 3 minutes and set aside.
3. Raspberry Jelly Filling:
4. Mix all the
5. Place in a pot and heat on medium.
6. Gently mash the raspberries and set aside to cool.
7. Donut Glaze:
8. Stir together the
9. Assembling:
10. Lay your chaffles on a plate and add the fillings mixture between the layers.
11. Drizzle the glaze on top and enjoy.

NUTRITION :

Calories per **Serving s** : 188 Kcal ; Fats: 23 g ; Carbs: 12 g ; Protein: 17 g

Oreo Keto Chaffles

Preparation time : 5 minutes

Cooking Time : 5 Minutes

Servings : 2

INGREDIENTS :

> 1 egg
>
> 1½ Tbsp unsweetened cocoa
>
> 2 Tbsp lakanto monk fruit, or choice of sweetener
>
> 1 Tbsp heavy cream
>
> 1 tsp coconut flour
>
> ½ tsp baking powder
>
> ½ tsp vanilla
>
> For the cheese cream:
>
> 1 Tbsp lakanto powdered sweetener
>
> 2 Tbsp softened cream cheese
>
> ¼ tsp vanilla

DIRECTIONS :

1. Turn on the waffle maker to heat and oil it with cooking spray.
2. Combine all chaffle ingredients in a small bowl.

3. Pour one half of the chaffle mixture into the waffle maker. Cook for 5 minutes.
4. Remove and repeat with the second half of the mixture. Let chaffles sit for 2-3 to crisp up.
5. Combine all cream ingredients and spread on chaffle when they have cooled to room temperature.

NUTRITION :

Carbs: 3 g;Fat: 4 g;Protein: 7 g;Calories:

Cinnamon Sugar Waffles

Preparation time : 5 minutes

Cooking Time : 12 Minutes

Servings : 2

INGREDIENTS :

2 eggs

1 cup Mozzarella cheese, shredded

2 tbsp blanched almond flour

½ tbsp butter, melted

2 tbsp Erythritol

½ tsp cinnamon

½ tsp vanilla extract

½ tsp psyllium husk powder, optional

¼ tsp baking powder, optional

1 tbsp melted butter, for topping

¼ cup Erythritol, for topping

¾ tsp cinnamon, for topping

DIRECTIONS :

1. Pour enough batter into the waffle maker and cook for 4 minutes.
2. Once cooked, carefully remove the chaffle and set aside.

3. Repeat with the remaining batter the same steps.

4. Stir together the cinnamon and erythritol.

5. Finish by brushing your chaffles with the melted butter and then sprinkle with cinnamon sugar.

NUTRITION :

Calories 8Kcal Fats: 16g Carbs: 4g Protein: 11g

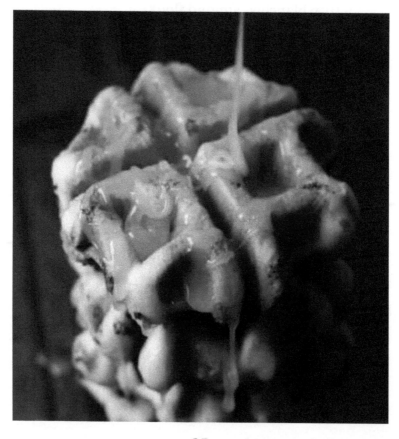

Cream Cheese Chaffles

Preparation time : 5 minutes

Cooking Time : 8 Minutes

Servings : 2

INGREDIENTS :

    2 teaspoons coconut flour

    3 teaspoons Erythritol

    ¼ teaspoon organic baking powder

    1 organic egg, beaten

    1 ounce cream cheese, softened

    ½ teaspoon organic vanilla extract

DIRECTIONS :

1. Preheat a mini waffle iron and then grease it.
2. In a bowl, place flour, Erythritol and baking powder and mix well.
3. Add the egg, cream cheese and vanilla extract and beat until well combined.
4. Put a portion of the mixture into preheated waffle iron and cook for about 3-minutes or until golden brown.
5. Repeat with the remaining mixture.
6. Serve warm.

NUTRITION :

Calories: 95Net Carb: 1.6gFat: 4gSaturated Fat: 4gCarbohydrates: 2.6gDietary Fiber: 1g Sugar: 0.3gProtein: 4.2g

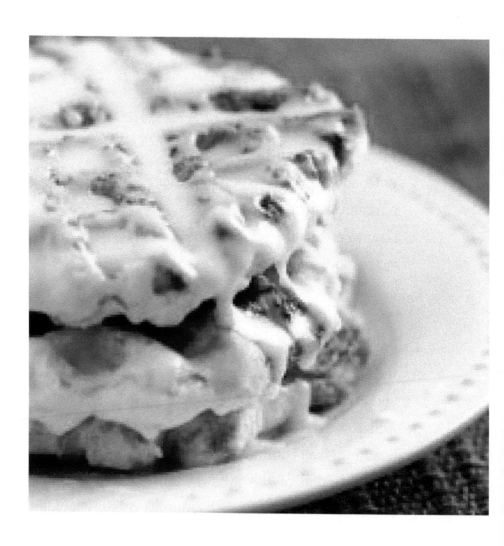

Mozzarella & Butter Chaffles

Preparation time : 5 minutes

Cooking Time : 8 Minutes

Servings : 2

INGREDIENTS :

    1 large organic egg, beaten

    ¾ cup Mozzarella cheese, shredded

    ½ tablespoon unsalted butter, melted

    2 tablespoons blanched almond flour

    2 tablespoons Erythritol

    ½ teaspoon ground cinnamon

    ½ teaspoon Psyllium husk powder

    ¼ teaspoon organic baking powder

    ½ teaspoon organic vanilla extract

DIRECTIONS :

1. Preheat a waffle iron and then grease it.
2. In a medium bowl, place all ingredients and with a fork, mix until well combined.
3. Put a portion of the mixture into preheated waffle iron and cook for about 5 minutes or until golden brown.
4. Repeat with the remaining mixture.

5. Serve warm.

NUTRITION :

Calories: 140Net Carb: 1.9gFat: 10.Saturated Fat: 4gCarbohydrates: 3gDietary Fiber: 1.1g Sugar: 0.3gProtein: 7.8g

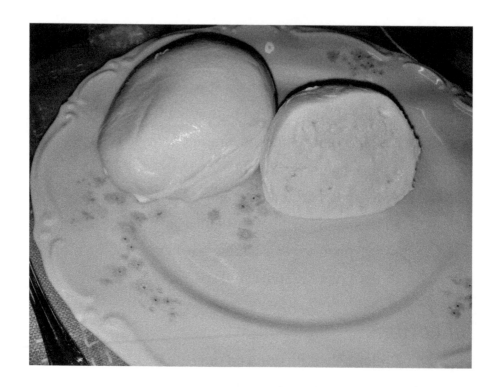

Pumpkin Pecan Waffles

Preparation time : 5 minutes

Cooking Time : 10 Minutes

Servings : 2

INGREDIENTS :

    1 egg

    ½ cup mozzarella cheese grated

    1 Tbsp pumpkin puree

    ½ tsp pumpkin spice

    1 tsp erythritol low carb sweetener

    2 Tbsp almond flour

    2 Tbsp pecans, toasted chopped

    1 cup heavy whipped cream

    ¼ cup low carb caramel sauce

DIRECTIONS :

1. Turn on the waffle maker to heat and oil it with cooking spray.
2. In a bowl, beat egg.
3. Mix in mozzarella, pumpkin, flour, pumpkin spice, and erythritol.
4. Stir in pecan pieces.

5. Spoon one half of the batter into the waffle maker and spread evenly.

6. Close and cook for 5 minutes.

7. Remove cooked waffles to a plate.

8. Repeat with remaining batter.

9. Serve with pecans, whipped cream, and low carb caramel sauce.

NUTRITION :

Carbs: 4 g;Fat: 17 g;Protein: 11 g;Calories: 21 0

Chocolate Cream Chaffles

Preparation time : 5 minutes

Cooking Time : 10 Minutes

Servings : 2

INGREDIENTS :

    1 organic egg

    1½ tablespoons cacao powder

    2 tablespoons Erythritol

    1 tablespoon heavy cream

    1 teaspoon coconut flour

    ½ teaspoon organic baking powder

    ½ teaspoon organic vanilla extract

    ½ teaspoon powdered Erythritol

DIRECTIONS :

1. Preheat a mini waffle iron and then grease it.
2. In a bowl, place all ingredients except the powdered Erythritol and beat until well combined.
3. Put a portion of the mixture into preheated waffle iron and cook for about 5 minutes or until golden brown.
4. Repeat with the remaining mixture.

5. Serve warm with the sprinkling of powdered Erythritol.

NUTRITION :

Calories: 7et Carb: 2.1gFat: 5.9gSaturated Fat: 3gCarbohydrates: 3.8gDietary Fiber: 1.7g Sugar: 0.3gProtein: 3.8g

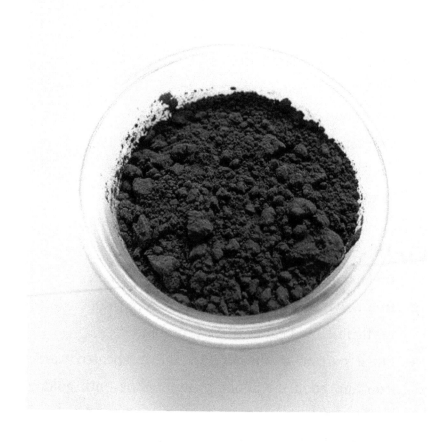

Blueberry Cinnamon Chaffles

Preparation time : 5 minutes

Servings : 3

Cooking Time : 10 Minutes

INGREDIENTS :

   1 cup shredded mozzarella cheese

   3 Tbsp almond flour

   2 eggs

   2 tsp Swerve or granulated sweetener of choice

   1 tsp cinnamon

   ½ tsp baking powder

   ½ cup fresh blueberries

   ½ tsp of powdered Swerve

DIRECTIONS :

1. Turn on the waffle maker to heat and oil it with cooking spray.
2. Mix eggs, flour, mozzarella, cinnamon, vanilla extract, sweetener, and baking powder in a bowl until well combined.
3. Add in blueberries.
4. Pour ¼ batter into each waffle mold.

5. Close and cook for 8 minutes.

6. If it's crispy and the waffle maker opens without pulling the chaffles apart, the chaffle is ready. If not, close and cook for 1-2 minutes more.

7. Serve with your favorite topping and more blueberries.

NUTRITION :

Carbs: 9 g;Fat: 12 g;Protein: 13 g;Calories: 193

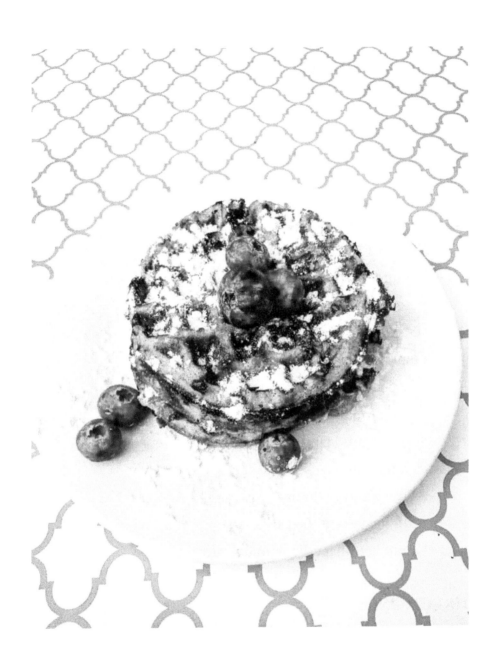

Gingerbread Chaffle

Preparation time : 5 minutes

Cooking Time : 5 Minutes

Servings : 2

INGREDIENTS :

 ½ cup mozzarella cheese grated

 1 medium egg

 ½ tsp baking powder

 1 tsp erythritol powdered

 ½ tsp ground ginger

 ¼ tsp ground nutmeg

 ½ tsp ground cinnamon

 ⅛ tsp ground cloves

 2 Tbsp almond flour

 1 cup heavy whipped cream

 ¼ cup keto-friendly maple syrup

DIRECTIONS :

1. Turn on the waffle maker to heat and oil it with cooking spray.
2. Beat egg in a bowl.
3. Add flour, mozzarella, spices, baking powder, and erythritol. Mix well.

4. Spoon one half of the batter into the waffle maker and spread out evenly.

5. Close and cook for minutes.

6. Remove cooked shuffle and repeat with remaining batter.

7. Serve with whipped cream and maple syrup.

NUTRITION :

Carbs: 5 g;Fat: 15 g;Protein: 12 g;Calories: 103

Chocolate Whipping Cream Chaffles

Preparation time : 5 minutes

Cooking Time : 8 Minutes

Servings : 2

INGREDIENTS :

    1 tablespoon almond flour

    2 tablespoons cacao powder

    2 tablespoons granulated Erythritol

    ¼ teaspoon organic baking powder

    1 organic egg

    1 tablespoon heavy whipping cream

    ¼ teaspoon organic vanilla extract

    1/8 teaspoon organic almond extract

DIRECTIONS :

1. Preheat a mini waffle iron and then grease it.
2. Add all ingredients in a bowl and beat them until well mixed.
3. Put a portion of the mixture in the preheated waffle iron and cook until golden brown, or around 4 minutes.
4. Repeat with the mixture that remains.
5. Serve it hot.

NUTRITION :

Calories: 94Net Carb: 2gFat: 7.9gSaturated Fat: 3.2gCarbohydrates: 3.9gDietary Fiber: 1.9g Sugar: 0.4gProtein: 3.9g

Almond Flour Waffles

Preparation time : 5 minutes

Cooking Time : 20 Minutes

Servings : 2

INGREDIENTS :

    1 large egg

    1 Tbsp blanched almond flour

    ¼ tsp baking powder

    ½ cup shredded mozzarella cheese

DIRECTIONS :

1. Whisk egg, almond flour, and baking powder together.
2. Stir in mozzarella and set batter aside.
3. Turn on the waffle maker to heat and oil it with cooking spray.
4. Introduce half of the batter into the waffle maker and spread it evenly with a spoon.
5. Cook for 3 minutes, or until it reaches desired doneness.
6. Transfer to a plate and repeat with remaining batter.
7. Let chaffles cool for 2-3 minutes to crisp up.

NUTRITION :

Carbs: 2 g;Fat: 13 g;Protein: 10 g;Calories: 131

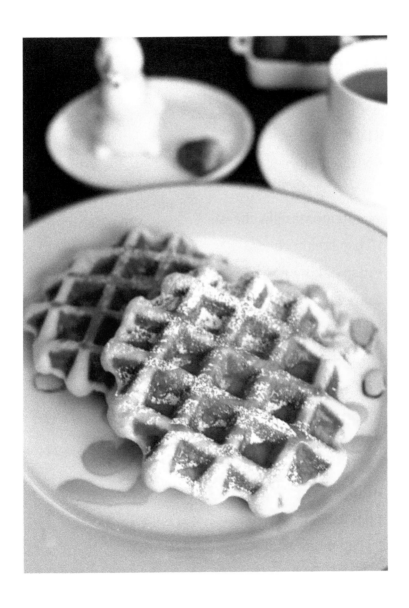

Strawberry cake Chaffles

Preparation time : 5 minutes

Servings : 1

Cooking Time : 25 Minutes

INGREDIENTS :

    For the batter:

    1 egg

    ¼ cup mozzarella cheese

    1 Tbsp cream cheese

    ¼ tsp baking powder

    2 strawberries, sliced

    1 tsp strawberry extract

    For the glaze:

    1 Tbsp cream cheese

    ¼ tsp strawberry extract

    1 Tbsp monk fruit confectioners blend

    For the whipped cream:

    1 cup heavy whipping cream

    1 tsp vanilla

    1 Tbsp monk fruit

DIRECTIONS :

1. Turn on the waffle maker to heat and oil it with cooking spray.
2. Beat egg in a small bowl.
3. Add remaining batter components.
4. Divide the mixture in half.
5. Cook one half of the batter in a waffle maker for 4 minutes, or until golden brown.
6. Repeat with remaining batter
7. Mix all glaze ingredients and spread over each warm chaffle.
8. Mix all whipped cream ingredients and whip until it starts to form peaks.
9. Top each waffle with whipped cream and strawberries.

NUTRITION :

Carbs: 5 g;Fat: 14 g;Protein: 12 g;Calories: 218

Cream Cheese & Butter Chaffles

Preparation time : 8 minutes

Cooking Time : 16 Minutes

Servings : 2

INGREDIENTS :

2 tablespoons butter, melted and cooled

2 large organic eggs

2 ounces cream cheese, softened

¼ cup powdered Erythritol

1½ teaspoons organic vanilla extract

Pinch of salt

¼ cup almond flour

2 tablespoons coconut flour

1 teaspoon organic baking powder

DIRECTIONS :

1. Preheat a mini waffle iron and then grease it.
2. In a bowl, place the butter and eggs and beat until creamy.
3. Add the cream cheese, Erythritol, vanilla extract and salt and beat until well combined.
4. Add the flours and baking powder and beat until well combined.

5. Place ¼ of the mixture into preheated waffle iron and cook for about 4 minutes or until golden brown.
6. Repeat with the remaining mixture.
7. Serve warm.

NUTRITION :

Calories: 202Net Carb: 2.Fat: 17.3gSaturated Fat: 8gCarbohydrates: 5.1gDietary Fiber: 2.3g Sugar: 0.7gProtein: 4.8g

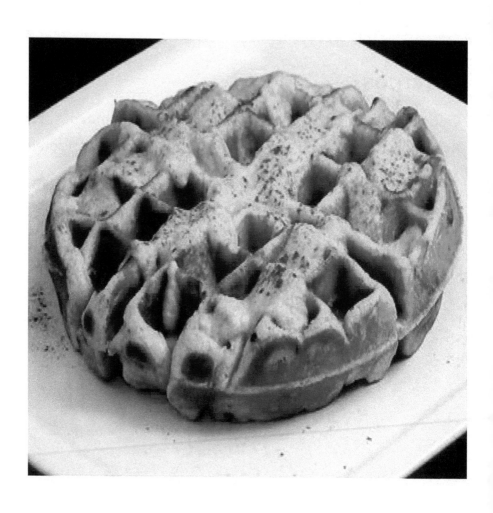

Chocolate Cherry Chaffles

Preparation time : 5 minutes

Servings : 1

Cooking Time : 5 Minutes

INGREDIENTS :

    1 Tbsp almond flour

    1 Tbsp cocoa powder

    1 Tbsp sugar free sweetener

    ½ tsp baking powder

    1 whole egg

    ½ cup mozzarella cheese shredded

    2 Tbsp heavy whipping cream whipped

    2 Tbsp sugar free cherry pie filling

    1 Tbsp chocolate chips

DIRECTIONS :

1. Turn on the waffle maker to heat and oil it with cooking spray.
2. Mix all dry components in a bowl.
3. Add egg and mix well.
4. Add cheese and stir again.
5. Spoon batter into waffle maker and close.

6. Cook for 5 minutes, until done.

7. Top with whipping cream, cherries, and chocolate chips.

NUTRITION :

Carbs: 6gFat: 1gProtein: 1gCalories: 130

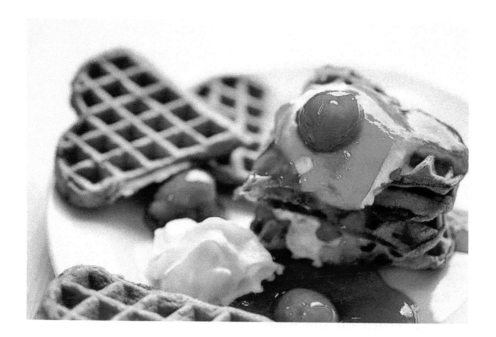

Coconut & Walnut Chaffles

Preparation time : 5 minutes

Servings : 8

Cooking Time : 24 Minutes

INGREDIENTS :

    4 organic eggs, beaten

    4 ounces cream cheese, softened

    1 tablespoon butter, melted

    4 tablespoons coconut flour

    1 tablespoon almond flour

    2 tablespoons Erythritol

    1½ teaspoons organic baking powder

    1 teaspoon organic vanilla extract

    ½ teaspoon ground cinnamon

    1 tablespoon unsweetened coconut, shredded

    1 tablespoon walnuts, chopped

DIRECTIONS :

1. Preheat a mini waffle iron and then grease it.
2. In a blender, place all ingredients and pulse until creamy and smooth.
3. Divide the mixture into 8 portions.

4. Place 1 portion of the mixture into preheated waffle iron and cook for about 2-3 minutes or until golden brown.
5. Repeat with the remaining mixture.
6. Serve warm.

NUTRITION :

Calories: 125Net Carb: 2.2gFat: 10.2gSaturated Fat: 5.2gCarbohydrates: 4gDietary Fiber: 1.8g Sugar: 0.4gProtein: 4.6g

Chocolate Chaffles

Preparation time : 5 minutes

Cooking Time : 10 Minutes

Servings : 2

INGREDIENTS :

¾ cup shredded mozzarella

1 large egg

2 Tbsp almond flour

2 Tbsp allulose

½ Tbsp melted butter

1½ Tbsp cocoa powder

½ tsp vanilla extract

½ tsp psyllium husk powder

¼ tsp baking powder

DIRECTIONS :

1. Turn on the waffle maker to heat and oil it with cooking spray.
2. Mix all ingredients in a small bowl.
3. Pour ¼ cup batter into a 4-inch waffle maker.
4. Cook for 2-3 minutes, or until crispy.
5. Transfer chaffle to a plate and set aside.
6. Repeat with remaining batter.

NUTRITION :

Carbs: 6 g;Fat: 24 g;Protein: 15 g;Calories: 296

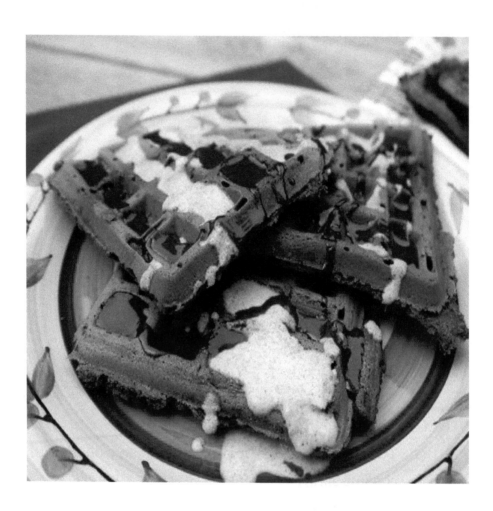

Chocolate Chips & Whipping Cream Chaffles

Preparation time : 5 minutes

Cooking Time : 8 Minutes

Servings : 2

INGREDIENTS :

    1 organic egg

    1 tablespoon heavy whipping cream

    ½ teaspoon coconut flour

    1¾ teaspoons monk fruit sweetener

    ¼ teaspoon organic baking powder

    Pinch of salt

    1 tablespoon 70% dark chocolate chips

DIRECTIONS :

1. Preheat a mini waffle iron and then grease it.
2. In a bowl, place all ingredients except for chocolate chips and beat until well combined.
3. Fold in the blackberries.
4. Put a portion of the mixture into preheated waffle iron and top with half of the chocolate chips.
5. Cook for about 3-4 minutes or until golden brown.

6. Repeat with the remaining mixture and chocolate chips.
7. Serve warm.

NUTRITION :

Calories: 110Net Carb: 1.Fat: 9gSaturated Fat: 5gCarbohydrates: 3.1gDietary Fiber: 1.3g Sugar: 0.2gProtein: 4g

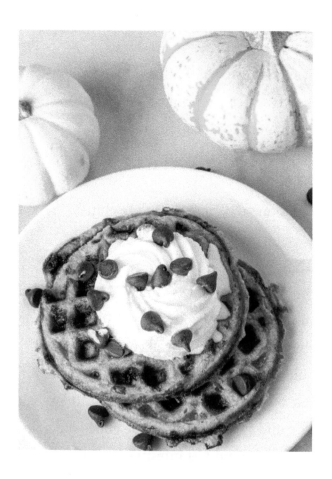

Spiced Pumpkin Waffles

Preparation time : 5 minutes

Cooking Time : 8 Minutes

Servings : 2

INGREDIENTS :

    1 organic egg, beaten

    ½ cup Mozzarella cheese, shredded

    1 tablespoon sugar-free canned solid pumpkin

    ¼ teaspoon ground cinnamon

    Pinch of ground cloves

    Pinch of ground nutmeg

    Pinch of ground ginger

DIRECTIONS :

1. Preheat a mini waffle iron and then grease it.
2. In a medium bowl, place all ingredients and with a fork, mix until well combined.
3. Put a portion of the mixture into preheated waffle iron and cook for about 4 minutes or until golden brown.
4. Repeat with the remaining mixture.
5. Serve warm.

NUTRITION :

Calories: 5et Carb: 1gFat: 3.5gSaturated Fat: 1.5gCarbohydrates: 1.4gDietary Fiber: 0.4g Sugar: 0.5gProtein: 4.9g

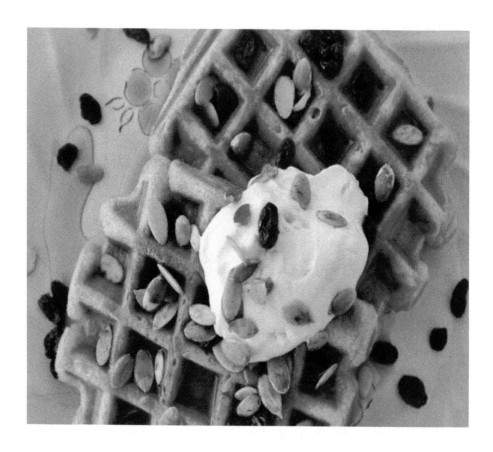

Vanilla Chaffle

Preparation time : 5 minutes

Cooking Time : 8 Minutes

Servings : 4

INGREDIENTS :

    2 tbsp butter, softened

    2 oz cream cheese, softened

    2 eggs

    ¼ cup almond flour

    2 tbsp coconut flour

    1 tsp baking powder

    1 tsp vanilla extract

    ¼ cup confectioners

    Pinch of pink salt

DIRECTIONS :

1. Preheat the waffle maker and spray with non-stick cooking spray.
2. Melt the butter and set aside for a minute to cool.
3. Add the eggs into the melted butter and whisk until creamy.
4. Pour in the sweetener, vanilla, extract, and salt. Blend properly.

5. Next add the coconut flour, almond flour, and baking powder. Mix well.
6. Pour into the waffle maker and cook for 4 minutes.
7. Repeat the process with the remaining batter.
8. Remove and set aside to cool.
9. Enjoy.

NUTRITION :

Calories per Kcal ; Fats: 27 g ; Carbs: 9 g ; Protein: 23 g

Preparation time : 5 minutes02

Banana Nut Chaffle

Preparation time : 5 minutes

Servings : 1

Cooking Time : 10 Minutes

INGREDIENTS :

1 egg

1 Tbsp cream cheese, softened and room temp

1 Tbsp sugar-free cheesecake pudding

½ cup mozzarella cheese

1 Tbsp monk fruit confectioners' sweetener

¼ tsp vanilla extract

¼ tsp banana extract

toppings of choice

DIRECTIONS :

1. Turn on the waffle maker to heat and oil it with cooking spray.
2. Beat egg in a small bowl.
3. Add remaining ingredients and mix until well incorporated.
4. Add one half of the batter to the waffle maker and cook for minutes, until golden brown.

5. Remove chaffle and add the other half of the batter.

6. Top with your optional toppings and serve warm!

NUTRITION :

Carbs: 2 g;Fat: g;Protein: 8 g;Calories: 119

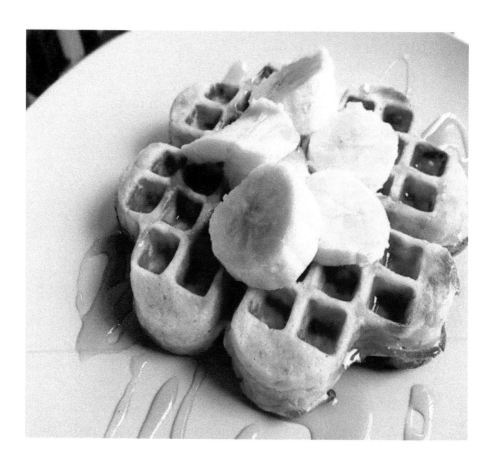

Chocolate Chips Pumpkin Waffles

Preparation time : 5 minutes

Servings : 3

Cooking Time : 12 Minutes

INGREDIENTS :

    1 organic egg

    4 teaspoons homemade pumpkin puree

    ½ cup Mozzarella cheese, shredded

    1 tablespoon almond flour

    2 tablespoons granulated Erythritol

    ¼ teaspoon pumpkin pie spice

    4 teaspoons 70% dark chocolate chips

DIRECTIONS :

1. In a bowl, place the egg and pumpkin puree and mix well.
2. Add the remaining ingredients except for chocolate chips and mix until well combined.
3. Gently, fold in the chocolate chips and lemon zest.
4. Place 1/3 of the mixture into preheated waffle iron and cook for about minutes or until golden brown.
5. Repeat with the remaining mixture.

6. Serve warm.

NUTRITION :

Calories: 9et Carb: 1.9gFat: 7.1gSaturated Fat: 3.3gCarbohydrates: 1.4gDietary Fiber: 2.6g Sugar: 0.4gProtein: 4.2g

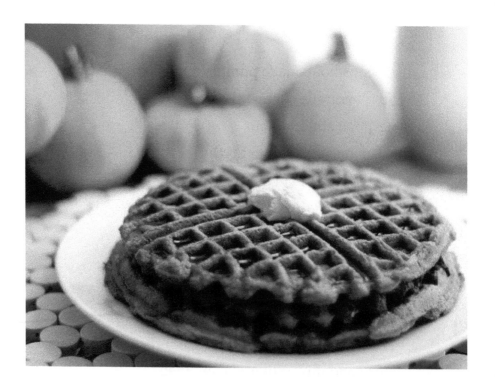

Oreo Chaffles

Preparation time : 5 minutes

Cooking Time : 5 Minutes

Servings : 3

INGREDIENTS :

Chocolate Chaffle:

2 eggs

2 tbsp cocoa, unsweetened

2 tbsp sweetener

2 tbsp heavy cream

2 tsp coconut flour

1/2 tsp baking powder

1 tsp vanilla

Filling:

Whipped cream

DIRECTIONS :

Introduce half of the mixture into the waffle iron. Cook for 5 minutes.

Once ready, carefully remove and repeat with the remaining chaffle mixture.

Allow the cooked chaffles to sit for 3 minutes.

Once they have cooled, spread the whipped cream on the chaffles and stack them cream side facing down to form a sandwich.

Slice into halves and enjoy.

NUTRITION :

Calories : 390 Kcal ; Fats:40 g ; Carbs: 3 g ; Protein: 10 g

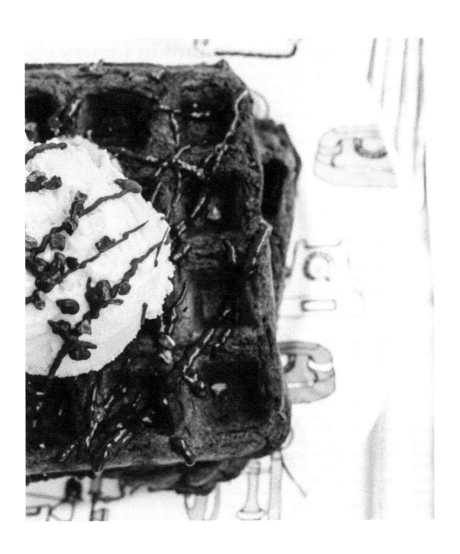

Whipping Cream Pumpkin Chaffles

Preparation time : 8 minutes

Cooking Time : 12 Minutes

Servings : 2

INGREDIENTS :

    2 organic eggs

    2 tablespoons homemade pumpkin puree

    2 tablespoons heavy whipping cream

    1 tablespoon coconut flour

    1 tablespoon Erythritol

    1 teaspoon pumpkin pie spice

    ½ teaspoon organic baking powder

    ½ teaspoon organic vanilla extract

    Pinch of salt

    ½ cup Mozzarella cheese, shredded

DIRECTIONS :

1. Preheat a mini waffle iron and then grease it.
2. In a bowl, place all the ingredients except Mozzarella cheese and beat until well combined.
3. Add the Mozzarella cheese and stir to combine.

4. Put a portion of the mixture into preheated waffle iron and cook for about 6 minutes or until golden brown.
5. Repeat with the remaining mixture.
6. Serve warm.

NUTRITION :

Calories: 81Net Carb: 2.1gFat: 5.9gSaturated Fat: 3gCarbohydrates: 3.1gDietary Fiber: 1g Sugar: 0.5gProtein: 4.3g

Chocolate Vanilla Chaffles

Preparation time : 5 minutes

Cooking Time : 5 Minutes

Servings : 2

INGREDIENTS :

½ cup shredded mozzarella cheese

1 egg

1 Tbsp granulated sweetener

1 tsp vanilla extract

1 Tbsp sugar-free chocolate chips

2 Tbsp almond meal/flour

DIRECTIONS :

1. Turn on the waffle maker to heat and oil it with cooking spray.
2. Mix all components in a bowl until combined.
3. Introduce half of the batter into the waffle maker.
4. Cook for 2-minutes, then remove and repeat with remaining batter.
5. Top with more chips and favorite toppings.

NUTRITION :

Carbs: 23 g;Fat: 3 g;Protein: 4 g;Calories: 134

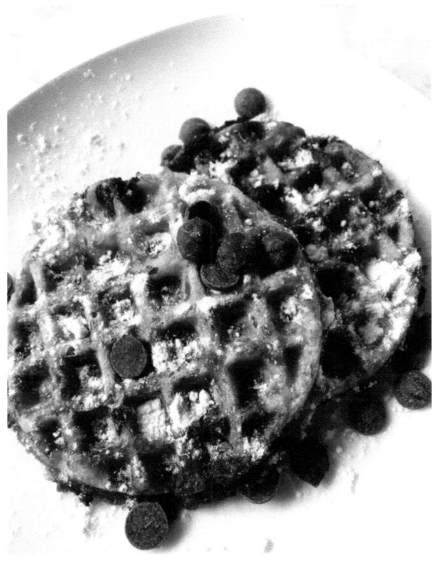

Churro Waffles

Preparation time : 5 minutes

Servings : 1

Cooking Time : 10 Minutes

INGREDIENTS :

    1 tbsp coconut cream

    1 egg

    6 tbsp almond flour

    ¼ tsp xanthan gum

    ½ tsp cinnamon

    2 tbsp keto brown sugar

    Coating:

    2 tbsp butter, melt

    1 tbsp keto brown sugar

    Warm up your waffle maker.

DIRECTIONS :

    Introduce half of the batter to the waffle pan and cook for 5 minutes.

    Carefully remove the cooked waffle and repeat the steps with the remaining batter.

Allow the chaffles to cool and spread with the melted butter and top with the brown sugar.Enjoy.

NUTRITION :

Calories per **Serving s** : 178 Kcal ; Fats: 15.7 g ; Carbs: 3.9 g ; Protein: 2 g

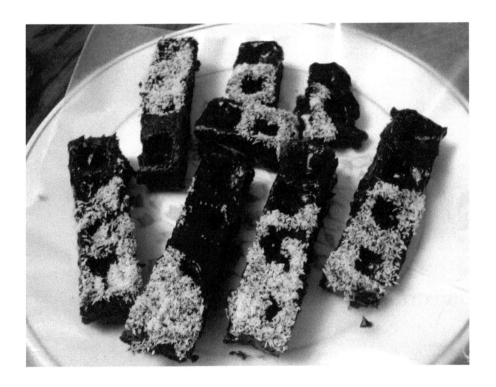

Chocolate Chips Lemon Chaffles

Preparation time : 8 minutes

Cooking Time : 8 Minutes

Servings : 2

INGREDIENTS :

2 organic eggs

½ cup Mozzarella cheese, shredded

¾ teaspoon organic lemon extract

½ teaspoon organic vanilla extract

2 teaspoons Erythritol

½ teaspoon psyllium husk powder

Pinch of salt

1 tablespoon 70% dark chocolate chips

¼ teaspoon lemon zest, grated finely

DIRECTIONS :

1. Preheat a mini waffle iron and then grease it.
2. In a bowl, place all **INGREDIENTS** except chocolate chips and lemon zest and beat until well combined.
3. Gently, fold in the chocolate chips and lemon zest.
4. Place ¼ of the mixture into preheated waffle iron and cook for about minutes or until golden brown.

5. Repeat with the remaining mixture.

6. Serve warm.

NUTRITION :

Calories: Net   Carb: 1gFat: 4.8gSaturated   Fat:
2.3gCarbohydrates: 1.5gDietary Fiber: 0.5g Sugar: 0.3gProtein:
4.3 g

Mocha Chaffles

Servings : 3

Cooking Time : 9 Minutes

INGREDIENTS :

> 1 organic egg, beaten
>
> 1 tablespoon cacao powder
>
> 1 tablespoon Erythritol
>
> ¼ teaspoon organic baking powder
>
> 2 tablespoons cream cheese, softened
>
> 1 tablespoon mayonnaise
>
> ¼ teaspoon instant coffee powder
>
> Pinch of salt
>
> 1 teaspoon organic vanilla extract

DIRECTIONS :

1. Preheat a mini waffle iron and then grease it.
2. In a medium bowl, place all **INGREDIENTS** and with a fork, mix until well combined.
3. Place 1/of the mixture into preheated waffle iron and cook for about 2½-3 minutes or until golden brown.
4. Repeat with the remaining mixture.
5. Serve warm.

NUTRITION : Calories: 83Net Carb: 1gFat: 7.5gSaturated Fat: 4.Carbohydrates: 1.5gDietary Fiber: 0.5g Sugar: 0.3gProtein: 2.7g

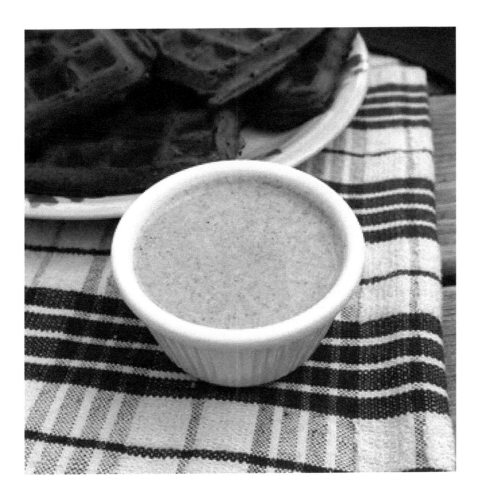

Carrot Chaffles

Servings : 6

Cooking Time : 18 Minutes

INGREDIENTS :

¾ cup almond flour

1 tablespoon walnuts, chopped

2 tablespoons powdered Erythritol

1 teaspoon organic baking powder

½ teaspoon ground cinnamon

½ teaspoon pumpkin pie spice

1 organic egg, beaten

2 tablespoons heavy whipping cream

2 tablespoons butter, melted

½ cup carrot, peeled and shredded

DIRECTIONS :

1. Preheat a mini waffle iron and then grease it.
2. Place the flour, walnut, Erythritol, cinnamon, baking powder and spices and mix well in a bowl.
3. Add the egg, heavy whipping cream and butter and mix until well combined.
4. Gently, fold in the carrot.

5. Add about 3 tablespoons of the mixture into preheated waffle iron and cook for about 2½-3 minutes or until golden brown.
6. Repeat with the remaining mixture.
7. Serve warm.

NUTRITION :

Calories: 165Net Carb: 2.4gFat: 14.7gSaturated Fat: 4.4gCarbohydrates: 4.4gDietary Fiber: 2g Sugar: 1gProtein: 1.5g

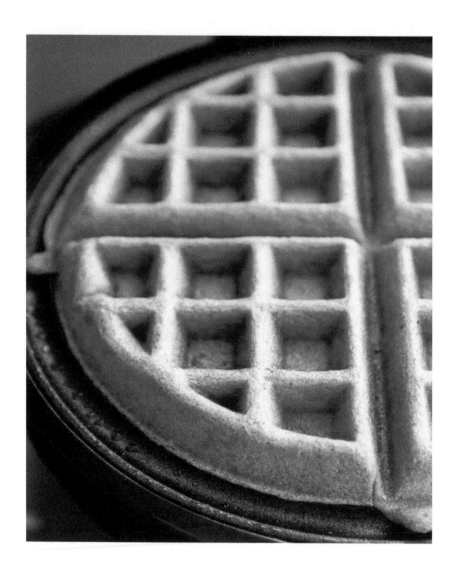

Yogurt Chaffles

Servings : 3

Cooking Time : 10 Minutes

INGREDIENTS :

½ cup shredded mozzarella

1 egg

2 Tbsp ground almonds

½ tsp psyllium husk

¼ tsp baking powder

1 Tbsp yogurt

DIRECTIONS :

1. Turn on the waffle maker to heat and oil it with cooking spray.
2. Whisk eggs in a bowl.
3. Add in remaining ingredients except mozzarella and mix well.
4. Add mozzarella and mix once again. Let it sit for 5 minutes.
5. Add ⅓ cup batter into each waffle mold.
6. Close and cook for 4-5 minutes.
7. Repeat with remaining batter.

NUTRITION :

Carbs: 2 g;Fat: 5 g;Protein: 4 g;Calories: 93

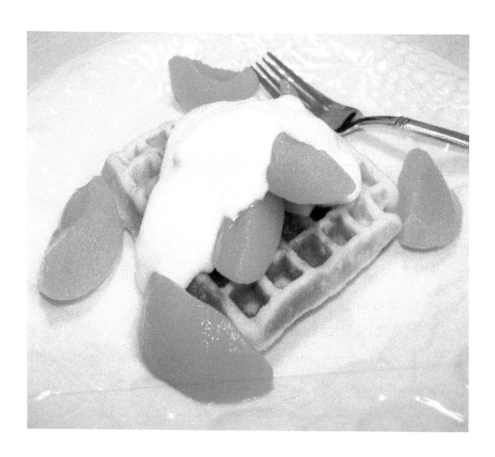

Chocolate Peanut Butter Chaffles

Preparation time : 5 minutes

Cooking Time : 8 Minutes

Servings : 2

INGREDIENTS :

    1 organic egg, beaten

    ¼ cup mozzarella cheese, shredded

    2 tablespoons creamy peanut butter

    1 tablespoon almond flour

    1 tablespoon granulated erythritol

    1 teaspoon organic vanilla extract

    1 tablespoon 70% dark chocolate chips

DIRECTIONS :

1. Preheat a mini waffle iron and then grease it.
2. In a bowl, add all ingredients except chocolate and beat until well combined. Gently, fold in the chocolate chips.
3. Put a portion of the mixture into preheated waffle iron and cook for about 4 minutes.
4. Repeat with the remaining mixture.
5. Serve warm.

NUTRITION :

Calories 214 Net Carbs 4.1 g Total Fat 18 g Saturated Fat 5.4 gCholesterol 84 mgSodium 128 mg Total Carbs 6.4 gFiber 2.3 g Sugar 2.1 gProtein 8.8 g

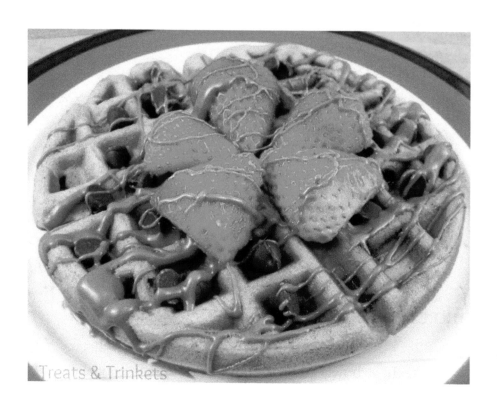

Ube Waffles With Ice Cream

Preparation time : 5 minutes

Cooking Time : 10 Minutes

Servings : 2

INGREDIENTS :

1/3 cup mozzarella cheese, shredded

1 tbsp whipped cream cheese

2 tbsp sweetener

1 egg

2-3 drops ube or pandan extract

1/2 tsp baking powder

Keto ice cream

DIRECTIONS :

1. Add in 2 or 3 drops of ube extract, mix until creamy and smooth.

2. Introduce half of the batter mixture in the mini waffle maker and cook for about 5 minutes.

3. Repeat the same steps with the remaining batter mixture.

4. Top with keto ice cream and enjoy.

NUTRITION:

Calories 65Kcal ; Fats: 16 g ; Carbs: 7 g ; Protein: 22 g

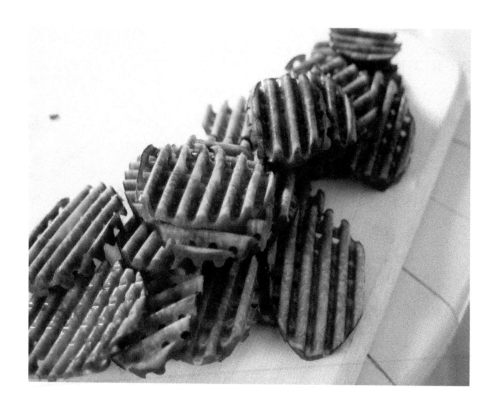

Berries Chaffles

Preparation time : 5 minutes

Cooking Time : 10 Minutes

Servings : 2

INGREDIENTS :

1 organic egg

1 teaspoon organic vanilla extract

1 tablespoon of almond flour

1 teaspoon organic baking powder

Pinch of ground cinnamon

1 cup Mozzarella cheese, shredded

2 tablespoons fresh blueberries

2 tablespoons fresh blackberries

DIRECTIONS :

Preheat a waffle iron and then grease it.

In a bowl, place the egg and vanilla extract and beat well.

Add the flour, baking powder and cinnamon and mix well.

Add the Mozzarella cheese and mix until just combined.

Gently, fold in the berries.

Put a portion of the mixture into preheated waffle iron and cook for about 4-5 minutes or until golden brown.

Repeat with the remaining mixture.

Serve warm.

NUTRITION :

Calories: 112Net Carb: 3.8gFat: 6.7gSaturated Fat: 2.3gCarbohydrates: 5gDietary Fiber: 1.2g Sugar: 1.Protein: 7g

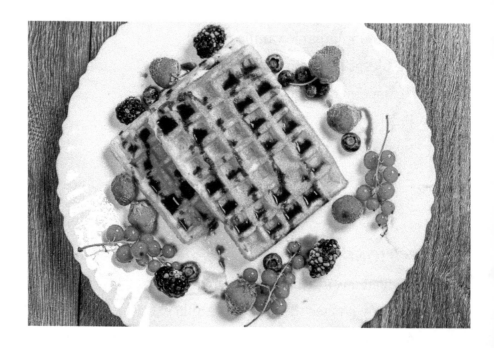

Cinnamon Swirl Waffles

Servings : 3

Cooking Time : 12 Minutes

INGREDIENTS :

For Chaffles:

1 organic egg

½ cup Mozzarella cheese, shredded

1 tablespoon almond flour

¼ teaspoon organic baking powder

1 teaspoon granulated Erythritol

1 teaspoon ground cinnamon

For Topping:

1 tablespoon butter

1 teaspoon ground cinnamon

2 teaspoons powdered Erythritol

DIRECTIONS :

1. Preheat a waffle iron and then grease it.
2. For chaffles: in a bowl, place all ingredients and mix until well combined.
3. For topping: in a small microwave-safe bowl, place all ingredients and microwave for about 15 seconds.
4. Remove from the microwave and mix well.

5. Place 1/3 of the chaffles mixture into preheated waffle iron.
6. Top with 1/3 of the butter mixture and with a skewer, gently swirl into the chaffles mixture.
7. Cook for about 3-4 minutes or until golden brown.
8. Repeat with the remaining chaffles and topping mixture.
9. Serve warm.

NUTRITION :

Calories: 87Net Carb: 1gFat: 7.4gSaturated Fat: 3.5gCarbohydrates: 2.1gDietary Fiber: 1.1g Sugar: 0.2gProtein: 3.3g

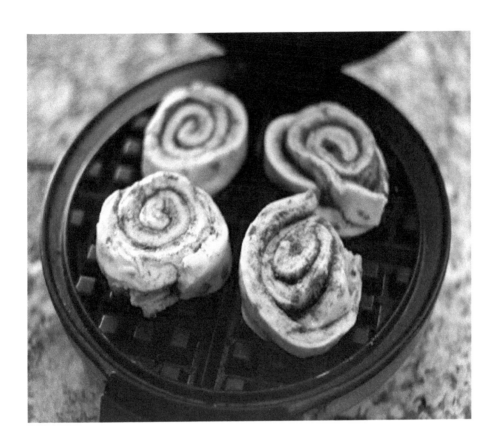

Chocolate Cream Cheese Chaffles

Preparation time : 5 minutes

Cooking Time : 8 Minutes

Servings : 2

INGREDIENTS :

　　　1 large organic egg, beaten

　　　1 ounce cream cheese, softened

　　　1 tablespoon sugar-free chocolate syrup

　　　1 tablespoon Erythritol

　　　½ tablespoon cacao powder

　　　¼ teaspoon organic baking powder

　　　½ teaspoon organic vanilla extract

DIRECTIONS :

1. Preheat a mini waffle iron and then grease it.
2. Add all ingredients in a medium bowl and, with a fork, mix until well mixed.
3. Put a portion of the mixture in the preheated waffle iron and cook until golden brown, or around 4 minutes.
4. Repeat with the mixture that remains.
5. Serve it hot.

NUTRITION :

Calories: 103Net Carb: 4.2gFat: 7.7gSaturated Fat: 4.1gCarbohydrates: 4.Dietary Fiber: 0.4g Sugar: 2gProtein: 4.5g

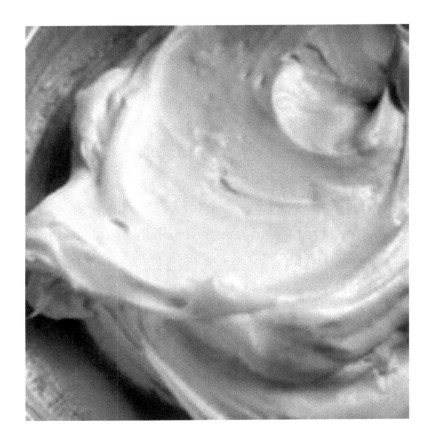

Colby Jack Chaffles

Servings : 1

Cooking Time : 6 Minutes

INGREDIENTS :

2 ounces colby jack cheese, sliced thinly in triangles

1 large organic egg, beaten

DIRECTIONS :

1. Preheat a waffle iron and then grease it.
2. Arrange 1 thin layer of cheese slices in the bottom of preheated waffle iron.
3. Place the beaten egg on top of the cheese.
4. Now, arrange another layer of cheese slices on top to cover evenly.
5. Cook for about 6 minutes.
6. Serve warm.

NUTRITION :

Calories 292 Net Carbs 2.4 g Total Fat 23 g Saturated Fat 13.6 gCholesterol 236 mgSodium 431 mg Total Carbs 2.4 gFiber 0 g Sugar 0.4 gProtein 18.3 g

Chaffle Birthday Cake

Preparation time : 8 minutes

Cooking Time : 16 Minutes

Servings : 2

INGREDIENTS :

Butter cream icing

Birthday Cake Chaffle:

3 tbsp cream cheese

1 tbsp almond flour

5 tbsp coconut flour

1 tsp baking powder

6 eggs

2 tbsp birthday cake syrup

DIRECTIONS :

Scoop 3 tbsp of the mixture into your waffle maker. Cook for 4 minutes and set aside.

Repeat the process until you have 4 cake chaffles.

Like a normal cake, start assembling your cake by placing one chaffle at the bottom as the base and adding a butter cream icing layer. Repeat the same process.

Pipe your cake edges with the icing and pile colorful shredded coconut at the center.

Once all the layers are completed, top with more icing and shredded coconut sprinkles.

Enjoy!

NUTRITION :

Calories per **Servings** : 390 Kcal ; Fats: 35 g ; Carbs: 18.9 g ; Protein: 11 g

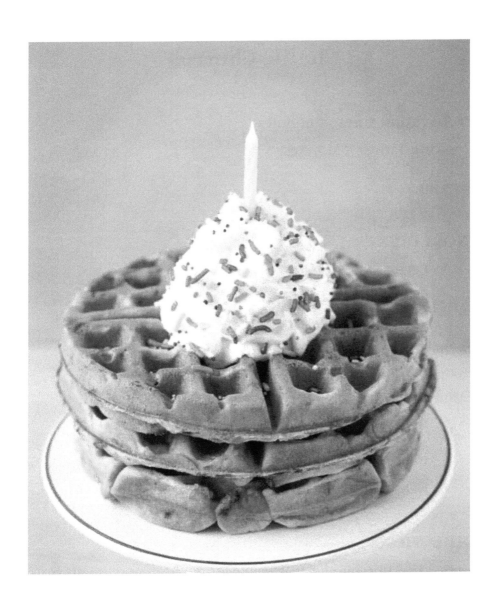

Chaffle Churros

Preparation time : 5 minutes

Cooking Time : 5 Minutes

Servings : 2

INGREDIENTS :

    1 egg

    1 Tbsp almond flour

    ½ tsp vanilla extract

    1 tsp cinnamon, divided

    ¼ tsp baking powder

    ½ cup shredded mozzarella

  1 Tbsp swerve confectioners' sugar substitute

    1 Tbsp swerve brown sugar substitute

    1 Tbsp butter, melted

DIRECTIONS :

1. Turn on the waffle maker to heat and oil it with cooking spray.

2. Mix egg, flour, vanilla extract, ½ tsp cinnamon, baking powder, mozzarella, and sugar substitute in a bowl.

3. Put a portion of the mixture into the waffle maker and cook for 5 minutes, or until desired doneness.

4. Remove and place the second half of the batter into the maker.
5. Cut chaffles into strips.
6. Place strips in a bowl and cover with melted butter.
7. Mix brown sugar substitute and the remaining cinnamon in a bowl.
8. Pour sugar mixture over the strips and toss to coat them well.

NUTRITION :

Carbs: 5 g;Fat: 6 g;Protein: 5 g;Calories: 76

Strawberry Chaffles

Preparation time : 5 minutes

Cooking Time : 8 Minutes

Servings : 2

INGREDIENTS :

  1 organic egg, beaten

  ¼ cup Mozzarella cheese, shredded

  1 tablespoon cream cheese, softened

  ¼ teaspoon organic baking powder

  1 teaspoon organic strawberry extract

  2 fresh strawberries, hulled and sliced

DIRECTIONS :

1. Preheat a mini waffle iron and then grease it.
2. In a bowl, place all ingredients except strawberry slices and beat until well combined.
3. Fold in the strawberry slices.
4. Put a portion of the mixture into preheated waffle iron and cook for about minutes or until golden brown.
5. Repeat with the remaining mixture.
6. Serve warm.

NUTRITION :

Calories: 69Net Carb: 1.6gFat: 4.6gSaturated Fat: 2.2gCarbohydrates: 1.9gDietary Fiber: 0.3g Sugar: 1gProtein: 4.2g

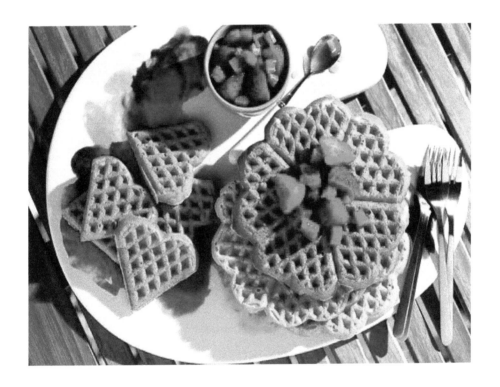

Lightning Source UK Ltd.
Milton Keynes UK
UKHW020634220621
385949UK00001B/65